Negative Calorie Diet & Dash Diet

LELA GIBSON

LELA GIBSON

CONTENTS

LELA GIBSON

LELA GIBSON

Negative Calorie Diet

Cookbook & Guide Which Will Help You To Burn Body Fat, Lose Weight And Live Healthy

Lela Gibson

LELA GIBSON

Introduction

I would like to thank you for buying the book, *"Negative Calorie Diet"*.

This book contains proven steps and strategies on how to burn body fat, lose weight and eat healthy.

Are you on the verge of giving up on your weight loss goals? Have you tried reducing your fat intake, eating fewer carbohydrates and all the diets that call for eating fewer proteins and carbohydrates, drank a lot of water, but you don't lose any weight? Does nothing seem to work?Well, I guess losing hope is understandable, but wait, DO NOT GIVE UP JUST YET! There is one more option, the best option in fact: *The Negative Calorie Diet.*

If we are to go by the facts, theNegative Calorie Diet is the fastest way to lose weight; you can lose up to 14 pounds a week when you adopt the diet! Thanks to this diet, losing weight is no longer a random dream or a hope; it is a reality for thousands of people across the globe.

In this book, you will learn more about the Negative Calorie Diet, how it works and some amazing recipes that will help you burn fat.

Thanks again for buying this book, I hope you enjoy it!

Negative Calorie Diet: What Is It

This unique diet draws upon theidea that some foodshave the 'negative calorie' effect that we ought to consider in burning fat. A food is considered to have a negative calorie effect when the calories these foods use to digest are typically higherthan the calories in the foods themselves.

When you eat something, you begin by chewing, a process that consumes energy. Some foods such as those higher in stringy fibers like celery will require more chewing, which will result in more energy expenditure, and there are otherslike pasta and cakes that don't require as much chewing.

After chewing, the foods go to the stomach through the esophagus and the other processes of digestion take over until absorption takes place and the body excretes the residual mass.

With negative calorie foods, this entire process uses up more calories than the foods have. The extra calories the body has to provide in order to process the foods are taken from the fat stores, and the more of these negative calorie foods you eat, the more your fat stores will lose calories, and as a result, the more fatyou will lose.

Let us take broccoli as an example: 100 grams (contains 25 calories).

When you eat 100 grams of broccoli, it takes your body about 80 calories worth of energy to digest it. This results in a net calorie use of 55 calories that should come from the fat stores in your body. As you can see, the 55 calories make up the negative net calorie.

Let us now take a counter example of a piece of cake containing 400 calories.

Your body will take about 150 calories to digest the piece of cake, leaving net 250 caloriesdeposited in the body and stored as fat.

The negative calorie diet consists of over 100 foods proven to have negative calorie qualities. Most of these foods are fruits and veggies that are high in fiber. Let us look at them in more detail in the following chapter.

Negative Calorie Food List

Here is a list of negative calorie foods:

Vegetables

Vegetables are highly nutritious and not high in calories when compared to many processed foods. Nonetheless, some vegetables are superior especially when it comes to the negative calorie food list. The following are vegetables you should consider including in your diet.

Artichokes	Bean sprouts	Broccoli	Cabbage	Cauliflower
Asparagus	Beets and beet greens	Brussels sprouts	Carrots	Celery
Chives	Cucumbers	Green beans	Mushrooms	Peppers (red, green, yellow)
Pumpkin	Sauerkraut	Spinach	String beans	Turnips
Corn	Eggplant	Lettuce	Peas	Pickles
Radishes	Scallions	Squash	Tomatoes	Zucchini
Garlic	Onion	Watercress		

Fruits

Just like vegetables, fruits are a healthier option and always the recommended healthy alternative to sugary foods. It is therefore a better idea to snack on a bunch of grapes than it is to snack on candy.

However, when it comes to fruit choices, you also need to make better choices because some fruits are high in calories; thus, not providing you the negative calorie effect you are looking for in negative calorie foods

The list below contains some good negative-calorie fruits you can eat:

Apples	Blackberries	Cantaloupe	Cranberries	Grapefruit
Honeydew melon	Lemons	Mangoes	Apricots	Blueberries
Cherries	Currants	Grapes	Kiwi	Limes
Nectarines	Oranges	Pears	Pomegranates	Strawberries
Watermelon	Peaches	Pineapple	Raspberries	Tangerines
Prunes				

Herbs and Spices

When it is a question of what you eat, even herbs and spices matter. Below is a complete list of herbs and spices you should always go for.

Chili pepper	Cloves	Ginger	Parsley	Cinnamon
Mustard seeds	Cayenne	Anise	Coriander/ Cilantro	Dill
Cumin	Fennel seeds			

Meat, Fish and Seafood

Red meat can be harmful to you, and many negative calorie diets don't recommend it; however, you do not have to avoid eating meat altogether, as it provides essential proteins and other nutrients. A good source of protein is fish for instance. Fish is lower in calories but high in essential nutrients like omega-3 fatty acids.

If you are allergic to fish, or if you are not a big fan of it, you can alternatively include small/reasonable potions of meat and chicken in your diet (I will teach you how in the recipes section).

The table below shows some of the best fish and seafood to include in your diet:

Clams	Crayfish	Mussels	Shrimp	Crab
Flounder	Tuna	Abalone	Buffalo fish	Cod
Terrapin	Bass	Catfish	Trout	

How To Make The Transition To Negative Calorie Diet

Now that you know what to eat, let us see exactly how you are going to be eating all that.

1. Make a smooth transition into the negative calorie diet so that you are comfortable with the entire process. Start by adding some negative calorie foods to the foods you normally eat in every meal in the 1:1 ratio. For instance, if having pasta with meatballs, you can serve 50% of this food and add chunks of zucchini to fill the other half.

You can also add a mixed salad to each meal you have; the salad should comprise of not less than 90% negative calorie foods. This means you have to look for ways to substitute any unwanted content such as any creamy high-fat substances with something like raspberry vinaigrette.

After some time, start slowly substituting the foods with the good (negative calorie) ones until your plate contains up to 90% negative calorie foods.

Note: We are only adding vegetables and fruits so far, not necessarily fully prepared negative calorie meals. Next, we will discuss the recipes so that you have entirely cooked meals too.

2.Use several vegetables to make a stir-fry. You can also make smoothie shakes with your favorite fruits including some berries. As said before, the negative calorie diet is largely a fruits and vegetables diet. However, this does not mean you should now start worrying about how you will survive as a vegetarian.

You can occasionallyenjoy small servings of chicken and some meat, and the recipes in the following chapter will reflect that. Nonetheless, the meats have to be in small amounts; remember, you are losing weight and so, you have to make some sacrifices.

First Thing to Do

Buy all the foods you think you require from the list, wash, cut them into bits then seal them in airtight containers for storage (in the fridge) so that you will have them handy anytime you need them. You do not want to come home from work tired in the evening without having a bunch of these foods readily available. If you do, you will be extremely tempted to grab something unhealthy.

If you are wondering whether you will be hungry on this diet plan, just know that you will not because these foods are filling because they are high in fiber as well as water; the perfect combination to be full.

Second Thing To Do

One thing you will discover as you start the negative calorie diet is that it is not easy to give up eating some foods. This is especially so if you've formed bad eating habits through the years. Habits such as eating in front of the television and snacking on junk food may be difficult to break. However, you have to do it.

This brings us to the second thing you need to do.

You need to get rid of foods that do not adhere to the negative calorie diet. As they say, out of sight, out of mind. Once you determine which foods to eat, the next thing is removing the foods that are not part of the diet. However, this does not mean that you need to get rid of such foods all at once.

Second Thing To Do

One thing you will discover as you start the negative calorie diet is that it is not easy to give up eating some foods. This is especially so if you've formed bad eating habits through the years. Habits such as eating in front of the television and snacking on junk food may be difficult to break. However, you have to do it.

This brings us to the second thing you need to do.

You need to get rid of foods that do not adhere to the negative calorie diet. As they say, out of sight, out of mind. Once you determine which foods to eat, the next thing is removing the foods that are not part of the diet. However, this does not mean that you need to get rid of such foods all at once.

As has been said, you should gradually shift to the negative calorie diet. You can't do this if you get rid of every food you should not eat. This means that you must determine how to go about doing away with such foods. Start by listing the foods down and then go about eliminating a few of the foods from your diet each week. This way, you will soon find yourself eating only the foods approved by the negative calorie diet.

Note: While on this diet, you should have no room for alcohol, sugar, or any sugar substitutes except stevia simply because sugar intake causes your body to produce more insulin. This hormone signals/tells the fat cells to pick up and convert any excess glucose into fat. Therefore, eating more sugar means more production of insulin and consequently, more deposits in the fat cells. We are trying to reduce fat in your body, not create more of it. In this regard, avoid all commercial dressings since most of them contain sugar and high fat content.

Third Thing To Do

The next step is to plan your meals. If you think about it, you usually have an idea of what you want to eat for breakfast, lunch and dinner. Unfortunately, you may have to stop eating many of those foods. This means you need to figure out what you will eat during meal times. This is where meal planning comes in.

Meal planning involves looking at your diet and determining which foods will go well together. When you are on the negative calorie diet, you find yourself enjoying a variety of fruits and vegetables. This is a nice opportunity to make different types of salads. Salads are easy to make and they contain many valuable nutrients. However, you can easily get bored if you eat the same type of salad day in, day out. This is why it makes sense to take a moment to plan your meals.

Meal planning is also quite useful when it comes to doing your shopping. As we have said, fruits and vegetables will feature prominently in your diet. You will want to use fresh produce as much as possible. This means you should time your shopping properly. If you determine which meals you'll be preparing beforehand, you can go ahead and shop for particular foods instead of shopping without a plan. This will ensure you have what you need when you need it.

Now that we have that out of the way, let us start cooking!

Negative Calorie Diet Recipes

While on a strict diet (such as this one), you might have a problem trying to decide what kind of dressing to use for your meals. Since I know it is important to be careful about what you are using, I will start by giving you two simple dressings that you will use on any meal you want.

Garlic and Herbs Dressing

Mix 1/2 cup of cold-pressed extra-virgin olive oil with juice from 1 lemon, 2 crushed garlic cloves and ¼ cup apple cider vinegar. Add some of your favorite negative caloriedried herbs such as parsley and cilantro.

This will yield 1 cup of dressing. Store the dressing in the fridge (for up to one month) to use on your foods.

Dijon and Yoghurt Dressing

For a delicious vegetable dip, mix Dijon mustard (2 tablespoons) with 2 cups low-fat yoghurt then add a pinch of chili pepper and a teaspoon of mixed dried herbs to spice it up.

Breakfast Recipes

Pumpkin Pancakes

Serves 4

Ingredients

1 cup of canned pumpkin

1 1/4 cups of water

2 teaspoons of cinnamon

2 cups Krusteaz pancake mix

1 egg, slightly beaten

1 teaspoon of baking powder

For the topping

1/4 cup of sliced pecans

5 tablespoons of pure maple syrup

Instructions

Combine all the ingredients for the pancake batter.

On a griddle or pan over medium heat sprayed with a little cooking spray, create a 10 cm circle of batter.

When the pancakes turn brown at the edges and you notice even bubbling across the top, flip them over to cook the other side.

In the meantime, toast pecans in a small pan until they turn slightly brown and give out the fragrance.

Serve with heated pure maple syrup.

Apple and Cinnamon with Almonds and Oat Bran

Serves 4

Ingredients

4 large apples

1 teaspoon of ground cinnamon

1/4 cup of oat bran

10 almonds, toasted and chopped

1 teaspoon of unrefined coconut oil

2 cups of unsweetened vanilla almond milk

2 packets monk fruit extract

Instructions

Wash the apples and cut into cubes.

Melt the coconut oil in a large nonstick skillet over medium high heat. Add the cinnamon and apples then cook for 2-3 minutes until the apples soften.

Remove from the heat, add almond milk, stir in the monk fruit extract and oat bran. Once mixed return back to the heat, stir, and bring to a simmer.

Cook for about one minute, until the mixture becomes thick and creamy.

Divide the mixture among four bowls then sprinkle each one with toasted almonds.

Negative Calorie Smoothie

Serves 2

Ingredients

5 strawberries

½ medium papaya

1 grapefruit

¼ cup ice

Instructions

Put all the ingredients in a blender; blend until smooth.

Serve and garnish with some strawberries and enjoy.

Lunch Recipes

Vegetable Soup

Serves 6

This is not your regular veggie soup; yes, it is simple, but it is full of negative calorie foods only.

Ingredients

6 cups of vegetable stock

1 cup of celery, diced

1 cup of green beans cut into about 1 inch pieces

1 medium zucchini, diced (approximately 2 cups)

1 cup small turnip, diced

1 jalapeno, seeded and finely chopped

1 medium onion, diced

1 cup of cauliflower florets

2 cups of shredded cabbage

3 cloves of garlic, finely chopped

2 cups of baby spinach

Salt and pepper to taste

Instructions

Mix the ingredients (except the spinach) in a pot, and bring to a boil.

Cover and let it simmer for 20 minutes.

Add the spinach, stir, and let it cook for one more minute.

Remove from the heat and serve.

Toast with Tomatoes

Serves 4

Ingredients

8 cups of spinach

½ ripe avocado, mashed well with a fork

Salt to taste

Freshly ground black pepper to taste

4 slices of natural gluten-free bread

4 (½-inch) slices ripe tomato

4 eggs, poached

Green hot sauce

Instructions

Place a nonstick skillet over medium high heat.

Add the spinach and cook until it wilts. Move the spinach to a colander and strain out as much water as possible. Put the now drained spinach in a bowl and season with green hot sauce and salt.

Use a toaster to toast the bread then season the avocado with salt. Evenly spreadthe pieces of avocado over each piece of toast then add a slice of tomato on top. Use pepper and salt to season the tomatoes and use the spinach mixture to top each slice evenly.

Place every piece of toast on a fresh plate. Finally, top with a poached egg and serve.

Meatballs with Mushroom Gravy

Serves 4

Ingredients

12 ounces lean ground beef

1 ounce Parmigiano Reggiano cheese, finely chopped

2 tablespoons arrowroot, dissolved in 2 teaspoons of stock

8 cups washed spinach

1 cup thinly sliced onion

4 cups sliced cremini mushrooms

Olive oil cooking spray

Freshly ground black pepper

Salt to taste

4 cups unsalted beef stock

1 cup finely chopped puffed brown rice

Instructions

Put the beef in a large bowl and push it to one side. Add rice and a cup of the stock to the other side of the mixing bowl; season with pepper and salt and allow the rice to absorb the stock for about 1 minute.

Mix the beef and rice using an electric hand mixture until well mixed. Taste and adjust the seasoning then use the mixture to form 16 meatballs.

Coat a skillet with olive oil cooking spray and place over medium heat. Once hot, put the meatballs and brown for one minute on one side. Turn and brown the opposite side for around 30 seconds and transfer to a plate.

Add the mushrooms to the skillet and sauté for a few minutes. Add the meatballs back to the skillet, then add the beef stock, arrowroot mixture, and cook until meatballs are cooked through.

Add the spinach and season with pepper and salt and cook until the spinach is wilted. Add the cheese, stir, and serve.

Dinner Recipes

Brussels Sprouts with Lemon and Almond Dressing

Serves 3-4

Ingredients

3 pints Brussels sprouts, shaved thinly

5 teaspoons of freshly minced garlic

Crushed red pepper flakes

1/2 cup of chopped fresh flat-leaf parsley

Salt

1 1/2 teaspoons of extra-virgin olive oil

1/4 cup of toasted almonds, finely chopped

1/8 teaspoon of ground cinnamon

1/2 cup freshly squeezed lemon juice

1 ounce of Parmigiano-Reggiano cheese, finely grated

Instructions

Place the Brussels in a large mixing bowl and place it aside.

Placea non-stick skillet over medium high heat then add the garlic and olive oil. Cook until the garlic turns deep golden brown. Remove from the heat then add the parsley, almonds, cinnamon, and red pepper flakes.

Return the skillet back to the heat sauté for about ten seconds.Remove from the heat, pour in the lemon juice, and then season with salt.

Add the dressing to the Brussels then toss well, add 75% of the cheese, and toss some more. Taste then add the seasoning and top with the rest of the cheese.

Chicken with Pesto

Serves 3 or 4

Ingredients

Water

6 garlic cloves, chopped

Dash of paprika

1 cup of fresh basil leaves

8 cups ofchopped escarole

Salt

1 ounce of Parmigiano-Reggiano cheese, finely grated

Olive oil cooking spray

Dash of cinnamon

Crushed red pepper flakes

1 small onion, thinly sliced

4 cups chicken stock,unsalted

12 ounces of skinless, boneless chicken breast sliced into 1/8 inch thick strips

Instructions

Pour 2 quarts of water in a medium pot and bring to a simmer. You will use this to poach the chicken.

Lightly coat a medium skillet with olive oil cooking spray then place it over medium high heat.

Add the garlic and cook until it turns golden brown. Add the cinnamon, basil leaves, red pepper flakes, onion, and paprika. Cook for roughly 2 minutes until the onion softens.

Add the escarole then cook until it is soft and wilted – for 2 more minutes. Add the stock, bring to a simmer, and then cover. Cook for about 5 minutes or until tender.

Add a pinch of salt to the simmering water and turn off the heat. Add the chicken and stir well until all parts separate. Cook until you notice the strips turning white (meaning they are half cooked). Use a slotted spoon to transfer the strips to a plate to cool.

Let the remaining mixture cook until most of the stock evaporates and looks like thick sauce or soup. Turn off the heat.

Add in half of the cheese, stir, and then season with salt to taste. Add the chicken strips then toss them to coat with the mixture and keep cooking until the strips have cooked enough through, for about 90 seconds.

Top with the remaining cheese, and then serve.

Vegetable Beef Soup

Serves 14

Note: This recipe has many ingredients and it is likely you will hate some vegetables or herbs. You can replace these vegetables and herbs with other ingredients on the negative calorie food list.

Ingredients

4 chopped onions

1 chopped red bell pepper

4 cups of sliced fresh mushrooms

10 chopped celery stalks with their leaves

2 cupsof fresh chopped broccoli

1 small chopped bunch of cilantro

5 box low sodium beef broth

1 large chopped green bell pepper

4 cups of chopped cabbage

6 large chopped fresh carrots

1 finely chopped head of garlic

6 cups of fresh chopped spinach

1 small bunch of Parsley

1 canof asparagus (drained)

2 cans of green beans (drained)

1 cupof canned artichokes (drained)

20 twists of cracked black pepper

1 tablespoon of Italian seasoning

Protein (you can use just about any meat preferably the fishes mentioned in the list)

2 10 oz. cans of tomatoes with green chili's (not drained)

2 cans of diced tomatoes with basil (not drained)

1/2 tablespoon of red pepper flakes

1 tablespoonof dried basil

2 small cans of chopped green chilies (not drained)

1 lb. 80/20 or leaner ground beef (drain if needed)

Instructions

Fill a large cooking pot halfway with the beef, chicken, or vegetable stock. Add all the canned ingredients while draining some as specified intothe pot.

Add water and all the spices then stir. Let it boil for some time, lower the heat to simmer for one hour or until the vegetables soften.

As the soup boils down, add some extra broth and stir.

Serve, garnish as desired, and enjoy.

Snacks

Apple Chips

Serves 2

Ingredients

2 large granny smith apples

1 teaspoon of stevia

1 teaspoon of cinnamon

Canola oil cooking spray

Instructions

Preheat your oven to 200 degrees.

Using a sharp knife, thinlyslice the apples crosswise. Arrange the slices on a single layer on a baking sheet then spray with canola oil cooking spray.

Evenlysprinkle the stevia and cinnamon over the apple slices.

Use the bottom third part of the oven to bake the apples until they are crisp and dry, roughly 2-2½ hours.

Alternatively, you could use a mastrad chipmaker. Not only is it easy and fast, you do not need the cooking spray. Just lay the apple slices on the chipmaker, sprinkle with cinnamon and stevia, and then microwave for 4-5 minutes.

Berry Salad

Serves 4

Ingredients

4 cups of mixed berries (blackberries, raspberries, blueberries, strawberries)

20 whole almonds, toasted and chopped

2 tablespoons of hemp hearts

1/4 cup of cooked quinoa

1 ½ tablespoons of fat free yoghurt

Instructions

Equally divide all the ingredients among four bowls and toss well to mix.

Fruit Salad

Serves 10

Ingredients

2/3 cup of fresh orange juice

1/2 teaspoon of grated lemon zest

2 cups of cubed fresh pineapple

3 kiwi fruits, peeled and sliced

2 oranges, peeled and sectioned

2 cups of blueberries

1/3 cup of fresh lemon juice

1/2 teaspoon of grated orange zest

1 teaspoon of vanilla extract

2 cups of strawberries, hulled and sliced

3 bananas, sliced

1 cup seedless grapes

Instructions

Add orange zest, orange juice, lemon juice and lemon zest, to a saucepan, place it over medium high heat, and bring to boil.

Decrease the heat to medium-low and let it simmer for 5 minutes. Remove from the heat and stir in the vanilla extract. Place it aside to cool.

Place the fruit in a clear glass bowl in layers starting with the pineapple, then strawberries, kiwi, bananas, oranges, then grapes and at the top, blueberries.

Pour the juice over the fruit layers then cover and leave in the fridge for 3-4 hours before serving.

Almond Cake with Berries

Serves 4

Ingredients

½ cup of almond meal

4 packets of monk fruit extract

1 teaspoon of vanilla extract

Olive oil cooking spray

2 eggs, separated; remove 1 yolk

3 tablespoons of raw coconut nectar

Salt

1 cup of mixed berries, mashed well with a fork

Instructions

Preheat your oven to 3750 degrees F.

Bake the almond meal until it becomes aromatic and well toasted –about 3-5 minutes. Remove from the oven and place it on a cool baking sheet.

Place the monk fruit and egg whites in a bowl and whisk until it forms stiff peaks. Use cooking spray to spray four paper cups. Using a toothpick or fork, poke holes in the bottom of each.

Place the almond meal into a mixing bowl then add the egg yolk, salt, vanilla, and coconut nectar. Fold the meringue into the mixture of almond and transfer the batter into the cups.

Place in the microwave and microwave for about thirty seconds. When the mixture has cooked through, place the cups on their sides and give them 45 seconds to cook.

Remove the cakes and place themupside down on four serving plates.

Get them off the cups and serve with berries.

Cucumber and salsa

Serves 2

Ingredients

2 cucumbers, peeled and sliced

12 garlic cloves, minced

¼ cup fresh cilantro, chopped

3 tomatoes, diced

½ sweet onion, diced

Sea salt and black pepper to taste

Instructions

Mix all ingredients except the cucumber in a bowl in order to make the salsa.

Place cucumber slices on a plate and serve with the salsa.

Negative Calorie Diet And Exercise: An Effective Way To Lose Weight Fast

I promised you some unique and cool exercise tips, right? Doing the following exercises will help you burn the fat much faster. All you have to do is to start slow and over time, increase the intensity, keep an open mind, and use the gym (for the ones that require it), where you have an instructor nearby.

Interval Training

This is all about high intensity exercises combined with short periods of rest. This will not only burn more calories than your typical cardio training, it will boost your body's ability to burn fat easily since it increases the production of the growth hormone, which is also a fat burning hormone, and adrenaline which assists in suppressing your appetite.

The intervals will work on your muscles, and help them use oxygen better so that your heart does not have to struggle to pump a lot to make them perform.

Do It!

Get on a treadmill or a stationary bike then use the guide below to start your own interval-training regimen:

Begin with a regular warm-up (any simple exercise to get your blood rushing). When done, run or pedal at a rate that is more than your regular cardio intensity by 20%. If you have never engaged in any serious cardio workouts before, you might want to check this first to understand what I am talking about.

After 30 seconds to 1 minute, reduce the intensity to a rate that is 50% less than the intensity of a regular cardio workout. Alternate the periods of 30 seconds to 1 minute of hard work with 30 seconds to 1 minute of relaxed pedaling or if you want, relaxed running for 6-10 intervals to finish your session.

As this gets simpler, increase each interval's intensity so that you work even longer during the difficult part, reduce your rest periods, or if you feel enthusiastic enough, add more intervals.

Repeat 3-4 times each week.

As you get the hang of this exercise, start the next:

Sprinting

Try sprinting up a hill since the impact on your joints will be much lower and can help you avoid injury. If there is no hilly ground in your area, try the alternative: the dag race approach. Start your sprint by increasing your speed from a jog.

To make the most of this exercise, keep the sprints short – ideally50 yards per sprint. This helps you sustain a high intensity all through and prevents injury.

If you want to increase the overall results of your sprint workout, increase your total number of sprints. This is better than going for long distance runs.

If you are new to exercising, do not do more than one workout per week. You can increase the days once you accustom to the exercise; just remember to allow at least two days of recovery between the workouts.

As you get the hang of the above exercise, start the next:

High Intensity Strength Intervals

Select two exercises that work different muscles completely or ones that use opposite movements. For instance, you can pair a pulling exercise with a pushing exercise or upper body exercise with a lower body exercise like pull-ups and squats.

For the latter, select a weight (if your instructor thinks you need one) with which you can do 10 repetitions. Alternate between the two exercises and do just five repetitions of each move in every set. Remember to rest between the sets so that you finish each set without failing.

Keep alternating between the exercises for a 10 or 15 minutes set time. Keep noting the total number of sets you can do. In subsequent sessions, try to beat your score by completing more sets in the same duration or completing the same number of sets but with heavier weights.

As you get the hang of the above exercises, start the next:

Countdown Workouts

Countdown workouts fit in the use of exercise pairs really well. They also keep you fully engaged in the exercises since you have to keep the count and pay attention.

With every round of the exercise pair, the training encompasses one lesser rep of each move; for instance, you move from a set of six to five...until zero.

You can also try density training where you pair opposing exercises for countdowns. For instance, kettlebell swing, pushups, and squat thrusts would work really well.

Do it!

Start by selecting your pair of exercises.

Perform six repetitions of the first exercise, then six reps of the other move. Go back to the first move and perform five reps then five more of the second exercise. Keep alternating until you reach zero.

In the subsequent workouts, add one rep to each exercise. If you want more countdowns, select a second pair from the list below, or just come up with your own pair of opposing moves.

Squat thrust, pushups

Kettlebell swing, squat thrust

Jumping jacks, pushups

Medicine ball side toss, medicine ball slam

As you get the hang of the above exercise, start the next:

Hurricane Workouts

This is essentially a workout protocol that entails lifting weights and interval training. We have three groups of exercises, called rounds in this type of workouts. Each round has an exercise that increases your heart rate, and a set of other exercises in between.

This design will allow you to keep your heart rate up throughout the workout (and burn significant amounts of calories) that typically lasts 16-22 minutes. Hurricane workouts have five levels and each one is an increased challenge. I have however prepared for you a sample routine you will work with below.

Note: This will require you to be more fit- if fit enough though, you can begin with this:

Warm up for the workout. For all rounds, do one set of each exercise and move on to the next exercise. Finish the whole round thrice before you move to the next round.

First round: Run on a treadmill at 10% incline, 10.5 mph for 25 seconds. Do a kettlebell Turkish getup about 4 times on each side of your body then 10 chin-ups.

Repeat this sequence thrice.

Second round: Run on a treadmill at a 10% incline, 11 mph for 25 seconds. Do 10 dips and a barbell rollout, 15 reps.

Repeat this process thrice.

Third round: Run on a treadmill at a 10% incline, 11.5 mph for 25 seconds. Perform the G.I row, 10 reps. Do the knee grab, 20 reps.

Repeat three times.

I need your help...

Thank you for buying this book!

I hope this book was able to help you to know more about the Negative Calorie Diet and how you can burn fat and lose weight with this diet, the next step is to put what you have learned into practice and actually adopt the diet if you want to see those pounds coming off.

Finally, if you enjoyed this book, then I'd like to ask you for a favor, would you be kind enough to leave a review for this book on Amazon? It'd be greatly appreciated!

I want to reach as many people as I can with this book, and more reviews will help me accomplish that!

If you have any questions or problems, please contact us: hello@freedomdestination.com

Thank you and good luck!

Dash Diet

Cookbook For Weight Loss With Action Plan And Easy Recipes

LELA GIBSON

INTRODUCTION

I want to thank you and congratulate you for buying the book, *"Dash Diet"*.

In an attempt to lose weight, we try almost any diet we can get our hands on. However, the sad thing is that most of these diets are just fad diets that don't offer long lasting results. It is important to point out that if you want to lose weight, you need to make a lifestyle change and not just adopting a diet for few days, losing a few pounds and gaining all that weight back after a while. This is why diets that are too restrictive are hard to adopt in the long run and this is where the DASH diet comes in.

The DASH diet is unlike any other diet because it focuses on lifestyle change rather than just losing a few pounds. Initially, the diet was started to help deal with high blood pressure; however, it is also quite effective in weight loss. The amazing thing is that it is not too restrictive and you can actually adopt it as a lifestyle. If you want to learn more about the DASH diet, what it entails and how you can use this diet to lose weight, this book will help you do just that.

In this book, you will learn more about the DASH diet, how it helps lower blood pressure and promotes weight loss, as well as some meal ideas, meal plans and recipes to get you started with the diet.

Thanks again for buying this book, I hope you enjoy it!

CONTENTS

What Is The DASH Diet?

The DASH (Dietary Approaches to Stop Hypertension) diet is an eating plan especially recommended for those with pre-hypertension or hypertension (high blood pressure). This diet helps in lowering blood pressure by availing key nutrients such as magnesium, calcium, and potassium all of which are associated with lower blood pressure. The DASH diet is rich in vegetables, fruits, nonfat dairy or low fat. It also includes lean meats, poultry and fish, whole grains, beans and nuts.

While the DASH diet was initially developed to help lower blood pressure, it is now also considered quite effective in weight loss, promoting hearth health, lowering inflammation and cholesterol.

Let us learn more about how this diet can do all the above:

Weight Loss

To lose weight, you have to create a calorie deficit. The DASH diet does not stress on calorie reduction; however, it recommends consumption of whole grains, vegetables, fruits and lean meats. Whole grains, fruits and vegetables are high in fiber, which is quite filling but relatively lower in calories. Meat, poultry, and fish being protein take quite some time to be digested; hence, you feel fuller for longer. If you combine this and reduce your intake of processed sugars, sweets and unhealthy fats, you will create a caloric deficit without too much work, which will lead to weight loss.

The great thing is that you will not feel hungry even as you lose weight because all the foods you will be eating are quite filling.

Lowers Blood Pressure

The DASH diet helps in lowering blood pressure due to its food composition. The DASH diet is rich in fiber, calcium, magnesium, and potassium; and has a low content of saturated fat and sodium. Adding more of these nutrients to your diet improves the electrolyte balance in your body thus allowing it to excrete the excess fluid that contributes to high blood pressure. These nutrients also reduce blood pressure by promoting the relaxation of blood vessels. Most people suffering from high blood pressure usually have these nutrients in deficiency so the DASH diet is quite effective at providing these nutrients; thus, lowering blood pressure.

Lower Cholesterol Levels

The DASH diet recommends intake of whole grains, which are high in fiber. Oats, brown rice, and whole-wheat products are excellent sources of fiber. Adequate fiber in your body has been shown to reduce cholesterol levels. Women should obtain 25 grams of fiber per day while men should aim for 38 grams.

Manages Insulin Resistance

The DASH is further favorable for those people with insulin resistance, pre-diabetes or diabetes as it helps in improving insulin sensitivity. The combination of nutrients and foods in the DASH diet may have an effect on various cellular targets that ultimately elevates changes in your body composition during weight loss thus effecting favorable impact on insulin action.

What To Eat And Avoid

As mentioned earlier, you should eat certain foods and avoid others while on the DASH diet. Let us look closely at the foods you can eat while on the DASH diet.

Foods To Eat

Vegetables: asparagus, artichokes, cabbage, mushrooms, bell peppers, cauliflower, beets, lettuce, onions, celery, broccoli, parsnips, Brussels sprouts, egg plants and corn

Fruit: apples, pineapples, blueberries, dates, kiwi fruit, papaya, mango, cherries, pears, apricots, plums, peaches, strawberries, honey dew, lemons, bananas, grape fruit, prunes, blackberries and tangerines

Non-fat or low fat dairy: Greek yogurt, low fat sour cream, feta cottage cheese, low fat buttermilk, mozzarella (part skim), chevre (goat cheese), soft parmesan cheese, low fat or fat free milk, trans fat free kefir, reduced-fat cheddar, Monterey jack

Lean proteins: fish fillets (plain), salmon, deli meat, turkey (skinless), chicken (ground, lean), shrimp, tofu, eggs, tempeh, beef: sirloin, round or flank and lean, pork

Whole grains: whole-wheat pasta, quinoa, amaranth, spelt, barley, wild rice, couscous, triticale, bulgur, kasha (buckwheat), millet, oats (old fashioned), and brown rice

Healthy snacks: bean-based spreads like black bean dip or hummus, raw veggie sticks and raw unsalted nuts, dried fruit popcorn, whole grain pretzels, whole grain crackers

Nuts and seeds: walnuts, sunflower seeds, pumpkin seeds, hazelnuts, cashews, almonds, nut butter

Beverages: sparkling water, herbal tea, low-sodium vegetable juice, 100% fruit juice, low-sodium broth

Foods To Avoid

The foods and drinks you should avoid while following the dash diet include foods high in salt and sugar as well as high fat snacks such as:

Canned soups

Sauces and gravies

White Bread and rolls

Cured meats and cold cuts

Processed Cheese

Salad dressings

Red meat that is not grass-fed

Pastries

Sugary beverages

Sodas

Salted nuts

Potato Chips

Cookies

Candy

With that information on the foods to eat and those to avoid, let us now learn how you can actually adopt the DASH diet.

DASH Diet Action Plan: How To Adopt The DASH Diet

You need to first begin by asking yourself what you will be eating, how to incorporate the DASH diet into your lifestyle, and what to do when you have to eat out among others things. The previous chapter mentioned the foods to eat and those to avoid; therefore, get rid of any food in the pantry or fridge that is not allowed on the DASH diet so that you don't give in to temptations.

Once you do this, stock up your kitchen with your favorite DASH diet allowed foods and snacks. To shop smart, create a shopping list for DASH allowed foods and carry it along with you when you go shopping. Also, use diet planning tools such as the daily DASH tracker and the weekly meal planner to plan your meals to avoid instances where it is time to eat and you don't have any clue as to what you should eat. Such scenarios are likely to lead to eating unhealthy foods, which will defeat the purpose of adopting the DASH diet.

Since the dash diet calls for a decrease in your sodium intake, below are ways you can use to reduce sodium intake:

- Learn the terms that indicate that a particular food is high in sodium such as broth, soy sauce, cured and pickled.

- Move away the saltshaker from where you are. "Out of sight, out of mind"

- Limit condiments such as pickles, catsup, mustard, and sauces that have salt-containing ingredients.

Sometimes, adopting the DASH diet can be quite difficult especially when you are used to eating unhealthy foods. In such cases, it is much better to slowly incorporate the allowed foods into your diet as you reduce the disallowed foods until you get used to the new foods because you stop eating the disallowed foods altogether. Below are effective ways of easily adopting the diet:

Slowly increase your intake of vegetables and fruits

The DASH diet plan recommends that you consume 4-5 servings each of vegetables and fruits each day for the standard 2,000-calorie diet. Therefore, if your plate is half full of simple carbohydrates and the other half is protein and vegetables, make an effort to ensure that vegetables are half of your plate with the other half being protein and your usual simple carbohydrates. Once you get used to eating more vegetables, you can then start eating complex carbohydrates.

To increase your fruit intake, instead of snacking on Potato chips, French Fries, a burger, some cookies, cake or candy, have a fruit instead. You can opt to have some berries, a slice of pineapple, mango, watermelon, or apple. You can also make a delicious smoothie with all your favorite fruits. The good thing is that the fruit will give you that sweetness that you may be looking for in high sugar snacks while still providing other essential nutrients. In addition, fruits are more filling and you are likely not to overeat on fruits as compared to cookies, which are very easy to overeat without providing any essential nutrients.

Incorporate a few servings of low-fat dairy products every day

Rather than completely avoiding high fat dairy products, incorporate the low-fat variety. Low-fat yogurt with some fresh fruit makes a great snack or breakfast option. You can also add milk and yogurt to homemade smoothies or even snack on an ounce of cheese with whole grain crackers or nuts. If you don't eat dairy products you instead can have non-dairy alternatives with minimal added sugar.

Switch starchy and sugary snacks for whole foods

The DASH diet eating plan doesn't leave you with much room in your calorie budget for traditional processed snacks such as cookies and chips. You need to select snacks that incorporate whole foods such as whole grains, low-fat dairy, nuts, fruits, and vegetables. Below are some friendly DASH-friendly picks:

1 cup edamame in the pod

1/4 cup unsalted nuts

Whole grain crackers with 1 ounce cheese

Veggies with hummus or bean dip

Plain, low-fat yogurt topped with fresh fruit

Celery sticks, banana or apple with 1 tablespoon nut butter

3- 4 cups air-popped popcorn

Limit red meat – choose poultry, fish, and beans instead

While red meat is allowed on the DASH diet, you should limit its consumption. Further, ensure that you eat grass-fed meat and not grain fed meat, which is high in saturated fat and omega 6 both of which contribute to obesity, high blood pressure and heart disease and promote inflammation. This is why red meat that isn't grass fed is not allowed on the DASH diet.

The DASH diet recommends 6 ounces of lean protein each day with fish, beans, and chicken being among the top choices. Most Americans eat plenty of poultry but most of them struggle with incorporating more beans and seafood into their diet. Load up on your legume intake by substituting canned, low-sodium beans for animal proteins in pasta dishes, chili, tacos, entrée salads, and hearty soups.

Plan your meals

The DASH diet lets you know what to eat and what to avoid. This makes it easier for you to plan your meals. Start by cataloguing the foods in your fridge and pantry. Next, determine which foods you need to purchase. This way, you can make your grocery list and determine which meals you will prepare during the week.

When planning your meals, it would be good to consider which foods are in-season. This is because in-season produce often tends to be cheaper, healthier and tastier. Some of the produce can be bought in bulk and frozen for later. If you intend to buy in bulk, you can make a practice of storing food in batches.

Why is this important?

Well, you can only eat 1-2 servings of food per meal. If you've prepared several servings and frozen the food together, you'd have to thaw the whole of it before dividing it and returning the leftovers to the freezer. This is not practical. On the hand, if you portion the food into zip-lock bags, you will only need to take the one you're going to use and leave the others for later.

Also, you need to make sure you label the food before freezing it for added convenience. This is because food can be 'forgotten' at the back of your freezer. Labeling the food shows you which foods need to be used before others. You should also make it a point to determine all the contents of your fridge at least once a month. This way, you'll know what you already have and what you need to buy.

Alternate your protein sources

Yes, you can eat proteins when you are on the DASH diet but this does not mean you have to get it from meat sources. The good news is that you can explore other sources of protein. You can eat things such as peas, lentils, beans and eggs. The important thing is to alternate your sources of protein.

Read labels

It only takes a few seconds of your time to read food labels and those few seconds can make a huge difference. As you become more conscious of your food choices, you will realize that similar products will vary when it comes to the amount of sodium and fat they have. You want to select low fat products and products that have reduced sodium. You can only make healthier choices by reading the labels.

Your choices matter

As you embark on the DASH diet, it will serve you well to remember that the choices you make will add up at the end of the day. If you are used to consuming appetizers, main courses and desserts for lunch and dinner, you will do well to monitor the foods you eat especially when it comes to the amount of sodium, calories and fat they contain. Remember, you are trying to cut back on sodium and to lose weight and reduce the bad cholesterol. Adding up the totals will put things into perspective.

When it comes to drinks, you will also want to be careful. For example, you know that drinking fresh fruit juice is healthier than drinking drinks such as soda. However, you must also keep in mind that fruit juice is high in carbs. Thus, it is better to drink such juices in moderation. If you drink them too much, you may end up gaining weight and that wil be counterproductive.

Truly, the DASH diet has many benefits. However, you need to make conscious food choices in order to reap those benefits. Once you embrace the diet, it will become part of your lifestyle. You will not only lose weight, but you'll also keep it off.

The following chapter will provide you with some ideas for DASH diet breakfasts, lunch, dinner and dessert as well as a 4-day meal plan.

DASH Diet Meal Ideas

Adopting a new diet is quite challenging especially when you are not quite sure where to start. In this chapter, I will give you some easy tips on how to change your meals and make the DASH diet friendly:

Breakfast

- When you are having scrambled eggs or omelet be sure to add chopped vegetables (broccoli, tomatoes, spinach, mushrooms)

- Instead of water, prepare oatmeal with low fat milk then top with a few nuts and sliced fruits

- Have a cappuccino or latte made with low fat or fat-free milk

- Pour yourself a bowl of whole-grain cereal along with low fat milk then add berries, banana slices, or dried fruit

- Make a breakfast parfait: layer granola or whole grain cereal, fruit and low fat yogurt in a tall glass

- Spread nut butter on whole grain toast then top with raisins, pear, apple and sliced banana

- Top ½ whole grain English muffin with a slice of low fat cheese and tomato sauce then place under the broiler for the cheese to melt

- For a quick smoothie, blend a banana or frozen fruit, 100% fruit juice and low fat yogurt

Lunch

- Instead of soda or any other soft drinks, drink low fat or fat free milk, sparkled water

- To prepare soup, use low fat milk instead of cream and water

- Top salads with pineapple chunks, seeds, crunchy nuts, dried fruits, grapes, mandarin orange sections and diced apples

- Enjoy broth based bean, lentil or vegetable soup or head for the salad bar

- Add extra vegetables such as grated carrots, mixed greens, peppers, and tomatoes to your sandwich

- Add extra frozen or fresh vegetables to canned or homemade soups

Dinner

- Begin your meal with a large green salad

- Grill or roast vegetables such as cauliflower, carrots, eggplant, mushrooms, zucchini, onions, and peppers and drizzle with balsamic vinegar

- Make one-pot meals with whole grains such as quinoa, buckwheat, bulgur, brown rice and barley; and peas or beans

- Stir-fry colorful vegetables then bite size pieces of tofu, shrimp, pork, or chicken with a bit of your desired stir-fry sauce

Dessert

- Fruit has always been natures perfect dessert – just sink your teeth into something that is juicy, sweet and in season:

- Try baked bananas, pears, or apples with a scoop of low-fat frozen yogurt

- Top low fat vanilla yoghurt with in-season, ripe berries and a sprinkle of sliced almonds

- For a tasty BBQ treat, grill fruit skewers over medium-hot coals

- Using berries, grapes, bananas, melon chunks and pineapple, create fruit kabobs

Below is a four-day DASH diet meal plan that you can adopt:

DASH Diet Meal Plan

Day 1

Breakfast: ½ cup (75 grams) of blueberries, 1 cup (90 grams) of oatmeal with 1 cup (240 ml) of skim milk

Snack: 1 medium apple

Lunch: mayonnaise and tuna sandwich made with 3 ounces (80g) of canned tuna, 1.5 cups (113g) green salad, 2 slices of whole grain bread, 1 tablespoon of mayonnaise, 1 cup (248g) vegetable soup

Snack: 1 medium banana

Dinner: 3 ounces (85g) of lean chicken breast cooked with ½ cup (75g) carrots, ½ cup (75g) broccoli and 1 teaspoon of vegetable oil. Served with 1 cup (190g) brown rice

Day 2

Breakfast: Scrambled eggs with vegetables, ½ cup (120 ml) fresh orange juice

Snack: 1 medium orange

Lunch: 3 ounces (85g) of lean turkey, ½ (38g) cup of green salad, 1.5 ounces (45g) low-fat cheese, ½ cup (38g) cherry tomatoes, 2 slices of whole wheat bread and 1 teaspoon of unsalted butter

Snack: 4 whole grain crackers and 1.5 ounces (45g) of cottage cheese

Dinner: 1 cup (200g) of mashed potatoes, ½ cup (75g) of broccoli, ½ cup (75g) green peas and 6 ounces (170g) of cod fillet

Day 3

Breakfast: 2 slices of turkey bacon, ½ cup (38g) of cherry tomatoes, 1 teaspoon of unsalted butter, 2 slices of whole wheat toast with a cup of tea made with skim milk

Snack: 1 cup Greek yogurt

Lunch: ½ cup (38g) of salad greens, 1 tablespoon of low-fat mayonnaise, ½ cup (38g) of cherry tomatoes, 1.5 ounces (45g) of low fat cheese and 2 slices of whole wheat toast

Snack: 1 cup of fruit salad

Dinner: Whole-wheat pasta and meatballs made with 4 ounces (115g) of turkey meatballs and 1 cup of pasta and ½ cup (75g) of green peas

Day 4

Breakfast: 1 cup (90g) oatmeal with ½ cup (75g) of blueberries, 1 cup (240 ml) of skim milk

Snack: 1 medium pear

Lunch: chicken salad made with 2 cups (150g) of green salad, 3 ounces (85g) of lean chicken breast, ½ cup (75g) of cherry tomatoes, 1 tablespoon of mayonnaise, ½ tablespoon of seeds

Snacks: 1 handful nuts

Dinner: 3 ounces of roast beef with ½ cup (75g) of broccoli and 1 cup (150g) of boiled potatoes.

I bet you are quite excited to get started with the diet. In the following chapter, we will look at some DASH diet recipes that you can try out.

DASH Diet Recipes

Breakfast Recipes

Vegetable Omelet

Yields: 4 servings

Ingredients

1/2 cup shredded reduced-fat sharp cheddar cheese (2 ounces)

1/8 teaspoon cayenne pepper

1/8 teaspoon salt

2 cups fresh baby spinach leaves or torn fresh spinach

8 eggs

2 tablespoons Italian (flat-leaf) parsley

Nonstick cooking spray

1 recipe Red Pepper Relish (see recipe at the end of whole recipe)

Directions

Use cooking spray to coat the inside of a nonstick skillet (10-inch) with flared sides. Heat the coated skillet over medium heat.

Combine the cayenne pepper, salt, parsley, and eggs in a large bowl. Use a wire whisk or a rotary beater to beat ingredients until frothy.

Pour the frothy mixture to the prepared skillet then immediately begin to stir the eggs continuously but gently with a plastic or wooden spatula until it looks like cooked egg surrounded by liquid egg. Stop stirring and cook until the egg is set but shiny for 30-60 more seconds.

Sprinkle the egg with cheese once it is set but still shiny. Top with ¼ cup of the red pepper relish and 1 cup of the spinach.

Lift one side of omelet and fold partially over filling using a spatula. Arrange the rest of the spinach on a warm platter then transfer the omelet to the platter.

Top with the remaining relish

Red pepper relish recipe

Combine ¼ teaspoon of black pepper, 1 tablespoon of cider vinegar, 2 tablespoons of finely chopped onion or green onion and 2/3 cup of chopped red sweet pepper

Tasty frittata

Yields: 4 servings

Ingredients

1 cup sweet cornfrozen

1 cup grape tomatoes, cut in half

1 cup sliced pepper strips

1 tablespoon diced fresh basil (or 1 teaspoon dry basil)

2 tablespoons canola oil

4 ounces shredded Jack/colby cheese or other cheese blend

6 eggs

1/4 cup sliced onion

Directions

Stir the eggs and basil in a small bowl.

Add the canola oil to a non-stick frying pan over medium heat. Once the oil is hot, add frozen sweet corn, onion, and pepper strips. (If desired, you may substitute a frozen mixture of onions and pepper strips).

Sauté the mixture for 3 minutes while stirring and turning over. Add the tomatoes and continue stirring and turning over. Cook for 5 more minutes until the onions become translucent.

Pour the egg-basil mixture onto the vegetables. Use a spatula to separate slightly in the interior or to lift the edges in order to allow the eggs to fall to the bottom of the mixture while the frittata cooks.

Top with cheese once the egg mixture has thickened all the way through then brown for 2-3 minutes under broiler.

Tip: ensure that you use a pan with metal handle since plastic is will most likely melt under the broiler. You could for instance try using an All-Clad pan.

Lunch Recipes

Tuna Sandwich

Yields: 1 serving

Ingredients

1 5 ounce can low sodium tuna packed in water, drained

1/3 cup cherry tomatoes, sliced

1/3 cup fresh arugula or other leafy greens

1/4 cup reduced fat whipped cream cheese

2 green onions, sliced

2 slices hearty multigrain bread

2 tablespoons extra-virgin olive oil

2 tablespoons fresh parsley, chopped

2 tablespoons freshly squeezed lemon juice

Black pepper

Directions

Add the tuna to a medium sized bowl and set aside. Add the green onion, pepper, parsley, lemon juice and oil in a separate bowl and whisk to combine. Pour 2/3 of your oil mixture into the bowl of tuna and mix well.

Coat both sides of the bread lightly with the remaining oil using a pastry brush or spoon. Grill the coated bread over medium high heat in a non-stick skillet until it is golden on both sides. Toss the remaining oil mixture with the arugula.

To assemble the tuna sandwiches: on each side of the grilled bread spread 2 tablespoons of cream cheese. Add ½ of the tuna mixture to each of the slices followed by ½ of the greens and finally top up with ½ of the cherry tomatoes.

Pork with Apples

Yields: 4 servings

Ingredients

1 1/2 tablespoons balsamic vinegar

1 1/2 tablespoons fresh rosemary, chopped

1 cup low-sodium chicken broth

1 pound pork tenderloin, trimmed of all visible fat

1 tablespoon olive oil

2 cups chopped apple

2 cups chopped onion

Freshly ground black pepper, to taste

Directions

Preheat your oven to 450 degrees F.

Use cooking spray to coat a baking pan lightly.

Heat olive oil in a large skillet over high heat then add the pork. Sprinkle pork with black pepper and cook for about 3 minutes until the tenderloin has browned on all sides then remove skillet from heat.

Transfer the pork to the prepared pan, put it in the oven, and roast the pork until a food thermometer indicates 165 degrees F (medium) for around 15 minutes.

Meanwhile, add the rosemary, apple, and onion to the skillet. Sauté for around 3 to 5 minutes over medium heat until the apples and onions are soft.

Stir in the vinegar and broth then increase heat and boil for about 5 minutes until the sauce has reduced.

To serve: place the roasted pork on a large platter then slice on the diagonal and place on 4 warmed plates. Top the pork with the apple-onion sauce and serve immediately

Dinner Recipes

Tuna and spinach sandwiches

Yields: 4 servings

Ingredients

2 ribs of celery, diced

2 tablespoons of olive oil

Juice of 1 lemon

8 slices 100% whole wheat sandwich bread

1/2 medium cucumber, peeled, seeded, and diced

1/2 teaspoon of dill weed

1 cup of fresh baby spinach

1/2 teaspoon of salt-free seasoning blend

1/2 small red onion, peeled and diced (about 1/4 cup)

1/4 teaspoon of freshly ground black pepper

1 6.4-ounce pouch of light tuna packed in water

Directions

Combine the dill weed, celery, onion, cucumber, and tuna. Drizzle tuna mixture with lemon juice and olive oil then stir. Season with the freshly ground black pepper and salt-free seasoning blend

Make the sandwich with ¼ cup of the baby spinach leaves and ½ cup of the tuna salad. Press down to compact the spinach and the tuna

Note: This recipe yields 2 cups of tuna that you can keep in the fridge for up to 3 days in order to make more meals.

Roasted Squash with Wild Rice

Yields: 6 servings

Ingredients

1 cup diced onion

1 small orange, peeled and segmented

1/4 cup chopped walnuts

1/4 teaspoon thyme

2 teaspoons canola oil, divided

1 cup fresh cranberries

4 cups cooked wild rice

1/2 tablespoon chopped Italian parsley

4 cups diced winter squash, peeled and cut into half-inch pieces

Black pepper to taste

Directions

Preheat your oven to 400 degrees F.

Add the squash to a roasting pan and toss with 1 teaspoon of oil.

Roast until brown for 40 minutes. Brown the onions in a hot sauté pan with the rest of the oil. Add the cranberries to the browned onions and sauté for 1 minute.

Add the rest of the ingredients and sauté until heated thoroughly for around 4 to 5 minutes

Serve.

Mushroom Chili

Yields: 4 servings

Ingredients

½ cup of sliced ripe olives

1 (19 ounces) can of white kidney beans(rinsed and drained)

8 ounces (about 2-1/2 cups) of sliced shiitake mushrooms

1 (14-1/2 ounces) can stewed tomatoes

1 ½ pounds (about 7-1/2 cups) of white button mushrooms, sliced

1 teaspoonof ground cumin

2 tablespoons of chili powder

1 tablespoon of minced garlic

1 cup of chopped onion

2 tablespoons of vegetable oil

Directions

Heat oil in a large sauce pan until hot then add the garlic and onion. Cook for about 5 minutes stirring frequently until the onions become tender.

Stir in the cumin and chili powder and cook for about 30 seconds until fragrant

Add the shiitake and white button mushrooms and cook for 6 to 8 minutes stirring occasionally until the mushrooms become crisp tender.

Add ½ cup of water, olives, beans, and stewed tomatoes. Simmer for about 10 minutes to blend flavors.

Serve with tortillas; garnished with shredded cheddar cheese, diced fresh tomatoes and shredded lettuce if desired.

Desserts

Oatmeal Walnut Cookies

Yields: 49 Cookies

Ingredients

1/2 cup chopped walnuts

1 cup bittersweet or semisweet chocolate chips

1 tablespoon vanilla extract

1 large egg white

1 large egg

2/3 cup maple syrup

4 tablespoons of cold unsalted butter, sliced into pieces

1/2 cup tahini (see Ingredient note)

1/2 teaspoon of salt

1/2 teaspoon baking soda

1 teaspoon of ground cinnamon

1/2 cup of whole-wheat pastry flour

1/2 cup all-purpose flour

2 cups of rolled oats

Directions

Position racks in the lower and upper thirds of the oven and preheat oven to 350 degrees F.

Line 2 baking sheets with silpat silicone liners or parchment paper.

Whisk the baking soda, rolled oats, salt, cinnamon, whole-wheat flour, and all-purpose flour in a medium bowl

Beat the tahini and butter in a large bowl using an electric mixer until the 2 ingredients are well mixed and form a paste.

Add the maple syrup and continue beating until ingredients are well-combined (note that the resulting mixture will be somewhat grainy)

Beat in the large egg followed by the egg white and finally the vanilla. Using a wooden spoon, stir in the oat mixture until just moistened. Stir in the walnuts and chocolate chips.

Roll a tablespoon of the batter into a ball with damp hands then place it on the prepared baking sheet. Flatten the batter ball slightly ensuring that the sides do not crack. Do this with the rest of the batter leaving a 2-inch space among the flattened balls.

Bake the cookies for about 16 minutes until golden brown switching the pans top to bottom and back to front halfway through.

Leave the cookies to cool on the pan for 2 minutes then move them to a wire rack to cool completely. Before baking another batch, leave the pans to cool for a few minutes. Store the cookies in an airtight container for up to 2 days. Freeze cookies for longer storage

Ingredient note: Tahini is a paste made from grinding sesame seeds. You can get it in some supermarkets and natural foods stores.

Chocolate Banana Cake

Yields: 18 Servings

Ingredients

2 cups all-purpose flour

1 large egg

1 teaspoon vanilla extract

1/2 cup Splenda Brown Sugar Blend

1/2 teaspoon baking soda

1 large ripe banana, mashed (1/2 cup)

1 egg white

1/2 cup semisweet dark chocolate chips

1/4 cup unsweetened cocoa powder

1 tablespoon lemon juice

3/4 cup soy milk

1/4 cup canola oil

Directions

Preheat your oven to 350°F.

Use nonstick spray to coat an 11 by 7 inch brownie pan.

In a large bowl, whisk together the baking soda, cocoa, brown sugar blend and flour

Whisk together the vanilla, lemon juice, egg white, egg, oil, soy milk and bananas in another bowl.

Make a hole in the middle of the flour mixture, and then pour in the chocolate chips and soy milk mixture.

Stir the ingredients together using a wooden spoon until well mixed then pour then spoon the batter into your prepared brownie pan

Bake for about 25 minutes until when you press the centre of the cake lightly with fingertips it springs back.

Snacks

Banana Smoothie

Yields: 2 servings

Ingredients

2 cups vanilla soy milk

1 banana, peeled

2 packets Splenda

1/2 avocado, pitted and peeled

1/4 cup unsweetened cocoa powder

Directions

Add all the ingredients to the blender and process until smooth then serve immediately

Blueberry Muffins

Yields: 12 muffins

Ingredients

1 cup low-fat milk

1 egg

1-1/2 cups whole-wheat flour

1/2 teaspoon baking powder

1/2 teaspoon salt

1/2 cup old-fashioned whole oatmeal (raw)

1/3 cup maple syrup

1/4 teaspoon baking soda

1/4 cup oil

2/3 cup frozen blueberries

Directions

Preheat your oven to 350 degrees F.

Use cooking spray to coat the inside of a muffin tin. Mix the dry ingredients (salt, baking soda, baking powder, oatmeal, and flour) in a bowl.

In another bowl mix all the other ingredients (egg, oil, milk, maple syrup). Pour the mixed wet ingredients onto the mixed dry ingredients then mix. Add the blueberries and gently stir; the resulting batter should be lumpy.

Scoop the batter into the muffin tins and bake until the muffins brown on the edges for around 20 minutes.

Serve warm or cool on a wire rack and store in the refrigerator in an airtight container.

I need your help...

Thank you again for buying this book!

I hope this book was able to help you to understand the DASH diet, why it is effective in lowering high blood pressure, how you can lose weight once you adopt this diet, what to eat, and the foods to avoid, how you can easily adopt the diet as well as some tasty recipes that you can try out. The next step is to take action NOW and adopt the diet because you can never know how great it is until you try it out.

Finally, if you enjoyed this book, then I'd like to ask you for a favor, would you be kind enough to leave a review for this book on Amazon? It'd be greatly appreciated!

I want to reach as many people as I can with this book, and more reviews will help me accomplish that!

If you have any questions or problems, please contact us: hello@freedomdestination.com

Thank you and good luck!

Preview Of '20 Easy And Fast Diet Tips For Losing Weight'

Before we start learning about the strategies you can use to lose weight, let's start by highlighting some of the benefits that will come as a result of shedding those extra pounds just to give you extra motivation to want to do something NOW.

Why You Need To Lose Weight

Healthy weight loss has over one hundred benefits; these include emotional and physical benefits. I will dedicate this section to discussing the health benefits that many people (and weight loss/health books) do not pay enough attention to.

1: You Avoid Pre-Diabetes or Type 2 Diabetes

Pre-diabetes/high blood glucose is a condition that develops when the blood sugar levels in your blood move past normal ranges but not enough to qualify as diabetes. When your body stops consistently producing insulin sufficient to meet your body's needs, or the amount produced does not work properly, type 2 diabetes is likely to develop. Being pre-diabetic places you at a very high risk of developing type 2 diabetes.

Being obese or overweight is a proven leading risk factor for type 2 diabetes because carrying excess weight typically makes it hard for cells to respond to insulin, and since the additional fat acts as an insulating layer, it makes it more difficult for the sugar to enter the cells, which results in more circulating blood sugar levels.

Nonetheless, if you are already a pre-diabetic, you can prevent the progression to diabetes by shedding some weight (to reduce the insulating layer on cells so that they respond more to insulin) and trying to maintain a healthy weight.

2: You Keep Your Heart Healthy

When it comes to heart disease, some of the key risk factors are high cholesterol and high blood pressure. Research shows that:

1. Excessive accumulation of body fat makes your body release particular chemicals that occur naturally into the bloodstream, which increases blood pressure, and

2. Being overweight makes the liver produce too much amounts of Low density Lipoprotein (LDL) also called cholesterol. LDL tends to be sticky and gathers in the walls of blood vessels, which causes the narrowing of arteries, a condition called atherosclerosis, which increases your risk of strokes and heart attack.

When you lose weight, your blood pressure often reduces and the liver naturally reduces the amount of LDL it produces.

Royal Adelaide Hospital conducted a research on cardiovascular improvements with respect to a special weight loss program. Their results showed a decrease of cholesterol by 12%, a 10% decrease of LDL, a 5% decrease in diastolic blood pressure, and an 8% decrease in systolic blood pressure.

Check out the rest of 20 Easy And Fast Diet Tips For Losing Weight on Amazon, go to:**http://amzn.to/2kGyXvc**

Check Out My Other Books

Below you'll find some of my other popular books that are popular on Amazon and Kindle as well.

Alternatively, you can visit my author page on Amazon to see other work done by me.

20 Easy And Fast Diet Tips For Losing Weight – An Easy-To-Follow Weight Loss Guide

Belly Diet: The Zero Belly Diet Step-By-Step Guide Which Will Help You To Lose Your Belly And Enjoy Your Flat Belly

Anti-Inflammatory Diet Guide – The Guide To Reduce Inflammation And Live A Healthy Life Without Pain

Clean Eating: Cookbook And Guide To Restore Your Body's Natural Balance And Eat Healthy

Negative Calorie Diet: Cookbook & Guide Which Help You To Burn Body Fat, Lose Weight And Live Healthy

Smart Fat: Cookbook With Fat Meals Which Help You To Lose Weight, Get Healthy And Improve Brain Function

9 781722 168773